YOUR KNOWLEDGE HAS VALUE

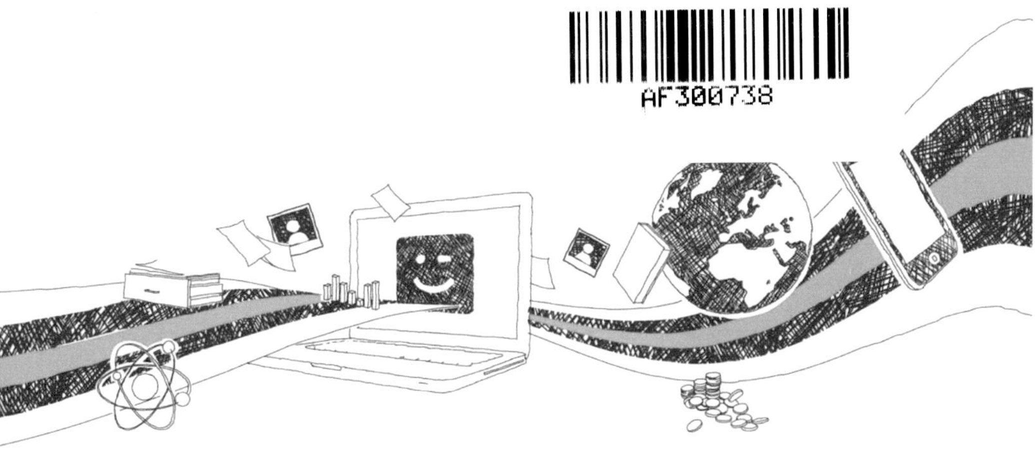

- We will publish your bachelor's and
  master's thesis, essays and papers

- Your own eBook and book -
  sold worldwide in all relevant shops

- Earn money with each sale

Upload your text at www.GRIN.com
and publish for free

Peter Okeke

Haematology Practice In Distressed Economy

GRIN Publishing

Bibliographic information published by the German National Library:

The German National Library lists this publication in the National Bibliography; detailed bibliographic data are available on the Internet at http://dnb.dnb.de .

Imprint:

Copyright © 2010 GRIN Verlag, Open Publishing GmbH
Print and binding: Books on Demand GmbH, Norderstedt Germany
ISBN: 978-3-640-80482-5

This book at GRIN:

http://www.grin.com/en/e-book/163508/haematology-practice-in-distressed-economy

HAEMATOLOGY PRACTICE IN DISTRESSED ECONOMY

BY

OKEKE PETER UBAH

2010

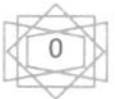

Chapter -1

Introduction

Types of laboratories

In most countries, there are likely to be some laboratories with limited resources, but in economic distressed countries, there are few laboratories with highly trained technologists and sophisticated equipment. In these countries therefore, i t is not unusual for laboratory tests to be carried out by nurses and ordelies in outpatient consulting rooms, corridors and in rural health centres.

Understaffing,poor morale, inadequate equipment and erratic supplies of reagents are chronic problems in laboratories in poorer countries and these factors have a major impact   on the range and quality of services that can be offered. Many smaller laboratories are multifunctional, performing Haematology, Parasitology, Clinical chemistry and Bacteriology tests. A blood transfusion service is usually available at the larger institutions and unless there is a national blood service, laboratory staff will be responsible for donor selection, blood collection and issuing of blood. If there is no organisation of public health laboratories, routine laboratories will be required to provide high quality health surveillance data for epidemiological and public health monitoring.

In a number of economically distressed countries, the difficulties are compounded by the fact that health services are becoming overwhelmed by expanding epidemics of HIV/AIDS(Human immunodeficiency vírus/Acquired immune deficiency syndrome), tuberculosis and malária. Diagnosis and monitoring of these diseases require a healthy,robust and reliable laboratory service. Thus malária diagnosis must be confirmed by a laboratory test because other disorders can masquerade clinically as malária. The diagnosis of tuberculosis may require boné marrow aspiration and culture and trephine biospy examination, especially in patients who are also HIV positive because in these cases sputum tests for acid fast organisms are frequently negative. Monitoring of HIV progression to AIDS and effectiveness of antiretroviral therapy requires Haemoglobin estimation, CD4-poistive lymphocyte counts and plasma viral load estimation.

The main purpose of this topic-(Haematology practice in distressed economy) is to point towards an effective haematology service that can be provided despite serious limitations. In planning such a service, it becomes imperative to identify what facilities are needed and to plan a network for referral when a clinical problem requires investigations beyond the facilities and expertise that are available locally. Thus, for example, successful management of haematological malignancies in countries with limited resources might involve the participation of local haematologists forming partinership with institutions in developed countries with consequent adaptation of standard protocols and improvement of local supportive care facilities.

Chapter-2

In a depressed economic countries, clinical laboratory services may be considered at three levels according to their size, staffing, and the work they undertake.

They are as follows:

A. Subdistrict facilities including health centres
B. District Hospitals
C. Central-regional and teaching Hospitals.

Level A….Subdistrict

The level A laboratory generally provides the means for helping to determine whether a patient should be referred to the local hospital. It may be simply a Haemoglobin estimation during the clinical consultation or it may be a side room where Basic laboratory tests are often carried out by nurses, assistants etc with no technical qualifications. The Haematology equipment available includes, a simple method of Hb estimation and a microscope for examination of slides for tuberculosis or maláría.

Level B…District Hospitals

District hospital laboratories are usually multipurpose performing bacteriological and biochemical as well as Haematological tests. Laboratory staff consists of one or two qualified technologists supported by assistants who often have little or no training. The minimum Haematology equipment includes,microscope,centrifuge and a simple colorimeter for Hb estimation.

Level C…Central and teaching Hospital

At this level the laboratory staff receives multidisciplinary training and each laboratory generally has a specialist technical head, whereas many of the more sénior staff will have received postgraduate training in their chosen discipline(for example, Haematology with Hospital transfusion practice or Bacteriology or Parasitology or Histopathology or Clinical Chemistry). Equipment generally includes;centrifuge,colorimeters, microscopes, Hb electrophoresis equipment and possibly blood bank centrifuges for the separation of blood components and Automated haematology analysers.

In many cases, these have been supplied by donor agencies, but long term funding to support maintenance and training for using these systems is often lacking and consequently they may be unreliable or not used at all owing to a shortage of appropriate reagents and inadequate maintenance and staff training.

AVAILABILITY OF TESTS AT EACH LEVEL

In a distressed economic countries, haematology tests that are available at the different levels of health care services are very variable and depend on local clinical needs, the equipment available, the number of laboratory staff and their technical skills. The following is a general

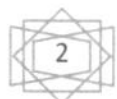

description of the tests that are likely to be required but all may not necessarily be available at the specified levels.

LEVEL A

HB estimation by simple method,Thin and THick blood films for malária screen, HIV serology tests supported by voluntary counselling and testing.

LEVEL B

A. Hb estimation

B. Blood film morphology, especially to identify the cause of anaemia.

C.Platelet and total white blood cell counts

D.Differential leucocyte count.

E. CD4 lymphocyte count

F. Malaria screening tests (thick and thin films) and rapid immunological test for plasmodium falciparium and others.

G. Screening test for sickle cell anaemia in prevalent áreas.

LEVEL C

In addition to tests carried out at level B, the haematology tests offered by level C might include the following;

A. Automated haematology anayzer for complete Blood Count
B. Hb electrophoresis or High performance liquid chromatography (HPLC)
C. HBA_2 and HBF determination
D. Glucose-6- phosphate dehydrogenase screen—by fluorescent spot or methaemoglobin reduction method.
E. Flow cytometry immunophenotyping
F. Polymerase chain reaction
G. HIV plasma viral load estimation
H. Bone marrow staining and assessment
I. Blood grouping and compartibility testing
J. Identification of blood group antibodies
K. Basic clotting testing(Thrombin test,Prothrombin test, Kaolin cephalin clotting time test or activated partial thromboplastin time test,fibrinogen assay and other factor assay tests,clotting time test and haemorragic time test)
L. Oral anticoagulant control
M. Blood component separation(plasma,packed cell and platelets,granulocytes etc)

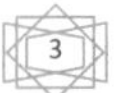

MICROSCOPES

In a distressed economic countries, microscope becomes the most important piece of equipment in the laboratory. It is necessary for the diagnosis anaemia, Tuberculosis, maláría and other blood parasitic infections or pathogens and for performing absolute and differential cell counts. Reliable assessment of these morphological features requires that the microscope is clean and correctly set with aligned lenses and inbuilt or reflected light to ensure clear images at high magnification. Failure to maintain the quality of microscopes to a high standard by routine maintenance and regular Professional servicing can lead to inaccurate diagnosis and inefficient use of the technologist time.

Chapter- 3

ESSENTIAL HAEMATOLOGY TESTS

Despite the relatively high cost of runing a laboratory service and the low per capita health care budget in distressed economic countries,there are very few data available on which to base rational decisions about essential haematology tests. In many of these countries, decisions for the laboratories are made at the central level by the health care planners whose interests are wider than those of the laboratory managers, but it is important to ensure that the viewpoint of the laboratory managers is respected. In deciding which tests are essential therefore, it is important to have reliable information concerning the clinical and public health needs of the local community to collaborate with the health providers or planners in projecting the médium and long term trends. The need for such information is especially urgent in countries where an overwhelming burden has been placed on the health services by the HIV/AIDS pandemic.

To ensure cost effectiveness of the laboratory services, tests with no proven values should be eliminated and new tests for which there is independent evidence of effectiveness should be introduced. For laboratories without Access to computerised data systems, an índex of realistic cost effectiveness can be obtained from the following formular, which takes account of various factors:

$$\underline{A \times 100 \times \mathbf{100}}$$

$$C \qquad B$$

Where A: cost per test, B:its diagnostic reliability and C: its clinical usefulness.

However, in laboratories with limited facilities these factors must be interpreted with caution because it is not possible to draw up a list of such tests that will be applicable to all countries or even to different regions within a country. The following aspects should be taken into account.

COST PER TEST

Often the cost of a test is calculated from the price of reagents divided by the number of tests performed. However, this oversimplifies the situation and is not accurate enough to form the basis for national policy decisions and budget allocation. When preparing a budget, the following formula provides a reasonably reliable estimate of the total annual costs:

$$[L \times N] + (C \times N) + E + M + O + S + T + A$$

Where L: labour costs for each test from estimate of time taken and the salary rate of each staff members performing the tests.

N: number of tests in the year

C: cost of consumables per test (including controls)

E: Annual equipment costs based on initial cost divided by expected life of the item

M: Annual maintenance and servicing of equipment

O: Laboratory overheads

S: Supervision

T: Transport and communication

A: Laboratory administration, including salaries of clerical and other non technical staff.

As an example of the effect of various factors on costs, in a typical district hospital laboratory in Africa, malária and tuberculosis microscopy comprised 22% and 46% respectively of the total number of tests performed, but when these factors are taken into account, tuberculosis smears actually accounted for 43% and malária microscopy for 9% of the overall laboratory budget.

DIAGNOSTIC RELIABILITY

The reliability of a quantitative test is defined in terms of the uncertainty of measurement of the analyte(sometimes referred to in documents as measurand). Diagnostic reliability is based on its accuracy and precision.

ACCURACY OF A TEST

Accuracy is the closeness of agreement between the measurement that is obtained and the true value; the extent of discrepancy is the systematic error or bias. This error can be eliminated or at least greatly reduced by using a referrence standard with the test, together with internal quality control and regular checking by external quality assessment.

PRECISION OF A TEST

Precision is the closeness of agreement when a test is repeated a number of times. Imprecision is the result of random errors; it is expressed as standard deviation(SD) and coefficient of variance(CV%). A test method may yield results that are precise but yet not accurate. Test results that are accurate and precise are desirable.

The quality of the test will influence its utility. However, the inaccurate test may result in a patient receiving inappropriate treatment. I t is also important to know the sensitivity and specificity of a test method.

DIAGNOSTIC SENSITIVITY OF A TEST

Diagnostic sensitivity is the proportion of patients with the disease who have a positive test results.It is defined by the number of TRUE POSITIVES(TP) divided by the sum of TRUE POSITIVES(TP) and FALSE NEGATIVES(FN), multiplied by 100. A diagnostic sensitive test should be used when a normal test results serves to rule out a suspected disease. A distinction must be made between diagnostic sensitivity and analytical sensitivity. Analytical sensitivity describes the lowest amount of a substance that can be detected accurately by a test method.

DIAGNOSTIC SPECIFICITY OF A TEST

Diagnostic specificity is the proportion of patients who are identified correctly by the test as not having the disease. It is defined by the number of TRUE NEGATIVES(TN) divided by the sum of TRUE NEGATIVES (TN) and FALSE POSITIVES (FP) multiplied by 100. A diagnostic specific test should be used when an abnormal results serves to confirm the presence of a disease. However, analytical specificity describes how well a test method can detect a particular substance rather than similar ones.

CLINICAL USEFULNESS OF A TEST

An assessment of the clinical usefulness of a test should be carried out by an independent clinician who is familiar with local diseases and the diagnostic support services that are available. This assessor needs to compare actual clinical practice with locally agreed- best practice- or, if available local guidelines. For example, transfusion guidelines may recommend that transfusions are given routinely to children with a Hb value of less than or equal to 4g/dl.

The assessor can record how many children with Hb below this level failed to receive a transfusion and how many transfusions were given without waiting for the Hb test results or na inappropriate Hb concentration. For each test, the assessor needs to judge whether it has been appropriately requested and is used to influence patient management or public health decisions.

MAINTAINING QUALITY AND RELIABILITY OF TESTS

Paradoxically, i t is in an economic distressed laboratories, where equipment and supplies are limited and training and supervision may be minimal, that the level of skills and motivation required to maintain quality of service need to be highest. Even the most Basic of laboratories should ensure that procedures are in place to monitor quality. In addition to monitoring the technical quality of each test, the quality of the whole services must be ensured both within the laboratory(internal control) and between laboratories(external control).

Standard operating procedures (SOP) should be drafted for every method. In addition to providing standardised techniques, these are excellent teaching resources and adherence to these procedures will drastically minimise errors.

QUALITY CONTROL OF A TEST METHOD (TECHNICAL QUALITY)

For a technical quality to be made, in every batch of tests, for example, of sickle cell screening tests, tests should include a known positive and negative samples. For monitoring constancy of Hb estimation, a high and a low value sample can be remeasured several times during the day.

INTERNAL QUALITY CONTROL (IQC)

Internal quality control is a system within an individual laboratory for ensuring that the whole test process, rather than just one technical element is of acceptable quality. Monitoring of quality by the use of controls that are put through the whole process and plotting a control chart will highlight problems with the system. For example, an inaccurate white cell differential count may point towards problems with sample collection and handling, slide preparation, fixing and staining, morphological interpretation and microscope quality as well as inadequate microscopy technique. Measures such as the introduction of standard operating procedures, inservice training, and equipment maintenance schedules are designed to improve performance and prevent problems.

EXTERNAL QUALITY ASSESSMENT (EQA)

Poor communication and transport facilities make it difficult to establish EQA in an economic depressed laboratories. Although participation in an international or a national or even local regional external quality assessment system may be beyond the capabilities of a small rural laboratory, it should be possible for them to link with neighbouring facilities. Rural laboratories can take advantage of programmes with established communications between the districts, to Exchange materials and results between different laboratories.

Such programmes might include district chief medical technologist´s supervisory visits or national vertical programmes such as tuberculosis monitoring or health education visits. A rural laboratory that detects a problem with its results needs to have a clearly defined reporting system to a higher level facility, which is in turn responsible for addressing the problem. Accreditation schemes either national or local can be set up to formally recognise laboratories that are performing well and to assist those that are not.

Chapter -4

BASIC HAEMATOLOGY TESTS

HAEMOGLOBINOMETRY

The most accurate method that may be available in distressed economic laboratories is the haemiglobin-cyanide (cyanmethaemoglobin) method. However, this requires a power source and considerable technical expertise to carry out accurate dilutions and to prepare the standard curve. Methods for measuring the Hb that are robust, accurate and can be used by unskilled health workers are mostly in use and are discussed below.

DIRECT READING HAEMOGLOBINOMETERS

HEMOCUE BLOOD HEMOGLOBIN SYSTEM

Hemocue blood haemoglobin system is a battery-or mains- operated portable, direct read- out machine that use disposable dry- chemistry cuvettes. It is precise and accurate (provided that only the specified cuvettes are used) and , unlike most other systems, it does not require predilution of the blood sample. Although the use of the unique disposable cuvettes makes this method relatively expensive, i t is very simple to use so that the cost may be offset by savings on training and supervision.

DHT HAEMOGLOBINOMETER

DHT haemoglobinometer is a portable, battery- or mains- operated, direct read-out machine. It has been specifically designed for use in poorer tropical countries. It uses a stable, inexpensive diluting fluid and has low power consumption. I t is simple to use because the diluted sample is placed in a cuvette that is inserted into the machine. This automatically initiates the reading and display of the haemoglobin value.

HAEMOGLOBIN COLOUR SCALE

Many colour comparison methods have been developed in the past, but these have become obsolete because the colours were not sufficiently comparable to blood or were not durable.However, the world health organization (WHO) has now developed a low-cost haemoglobin colour scale for anaemia screening test where there is no laboratory. It consists of a set of printed colour shades representing haemoglobin levels between 4g/dl to 14g/dl. The colour of a drop of blood collected into a specific type of matrix is compared to that on the chart. It is intended for detecting the presence of anaemia and estimating its severity in 2g/dl(20g/l) increments.

The utility of the scale in clinical practice has been demonstrated by field trials in rural antenatal clinics and peripheral health centres. However, care must be taken to follow the instructions exactly because poor lighting, allowing the blood spot to dry out and using the incorrect type of matrix for the test strips can have detrimental effects on the results.

PACKED CELL VOLUME (PCV)

Although,the packed cell volume can be used as a simple screen for anaemia and as a rough guide to the accuracy of haemoglobin measurements,i t is not a substitute for a well performed haemoglobin estimation. In addition to the technical problems, PCV has particular problems in economically distressed settings that may lead to errors in estimating it. The lack of a mechanical mixing device means that specimens may not be adequately mixed. A lack of high quality sealant for the microhaematocrit tubes means that they often leak during centrifugation. Because the microhaematocrit tubes are difficult to label, samples may get mixed up in the centrifuge, especially when pressure of work is high and there is lack of supervision. Erratic power supplies, lack of devices for measuring –g—forces and poor equipment maintenance, results in inadequate centrifugation with incomplete packing of the red cells.

MANUAL CELL COUNTS USING COUNTING CHAMBERS

Visual counting of blood cells is an acceptable alternative to electronic counting systems for white blood cell count and platelet cell count. It is not recommended for routine red blood cell counts because the number of blood cells that can be counted within a reasonable time in the routine laboratory (for example about 400 cells) will be too few to ensure a sufficiently precise results.

COUNTING CHAMBERS

The visibility of the rulings in the counting chambers is as important as the accuracy of calibration, so that chambers with a metallised surface and Neubauer or improved Neubauer rulings are recommended. These have nine 1mm× 1mm ruled áreas, which when covered correctly with the special thick coverglass, each contain a volume of 0.1μL of diluted blood sample. Coverslips designed for mounting of microscopy preparations must not be used with counting chambers.

The sample is introduced between the chamber and the coverslip using a pipette or capillary tube and the preparation is examined using a 40× objective and ×6 or×10 eyepieces under the microscope after few minutes to allow the cells to settle. With Neubauer or improved Neubauer counting chambers, count the cells in 4 or 8 horizontal rectangles of 1mm × 0.05mm (80 or 160 small squares) or in 5 or 10 groups of 16 small squares, including the cells that touch the bottom and left hand margins of the small squares.

TOTAL WHITE BLOOD CELL COUNT

To make the counting of white cells easier, diluted whole blood is mixed with a fluid to lyse the red cells and staining the white cell nuclei deep violet – black.

METHOD

Make a 1 in 20 dilution of blood by adding 0.1ml of well mixed blood to 1.9ml of turks solution in a small glass tube, mix at least for 2 minutes. Fill a clean dry counting chamber with its coverslips already in place without delay, allow for few minutes. This is simply accomplished with the aid of a plastic Pasteur pipette or a length of stout capillary glass tubing that has been allowed to take up the suspension by capillarity. Take care that the counting chamber is filled in one action and that no fluid flows into the surrounding moat. Leave the chamber undisturbed on a bench for at least 2 minutes for the cells to settle, but not much longer because drying at the edges of the preparation iniates currents that cause movement of the cells after they have settled. The bench must be free of vibrations, and the chamber must not be exposed to draughts or to direct sunlight or other sources of heat. Count the cells using ×10 objective in the entire área made for counting. Express results by multiplication of the number of cells counted by a factor 50. For example, cells counted in total is 110 cells,therefore (110 cells ×50)=5.500 mm^3

HOW TO PERFORM WHITE CELL ESTIMATE

❖ Scan thin área using the oil immersion lens
❖ Observe 10 fields, counting all white cells in each field
❖ Average the number of white cells seen per oil immersion field.

Multiply the number of wbcs/oil immersion field by 3000 and compare results with wbcs count with chamber.

PLATELET COUNT

Platelets are adhesive to foreign objects and to each other which makes it difficult to count them.They are also small and could be confused easily with dirt. It is advisable to use PHASE CONTRAST MICROSCOPY to count platelets for accuracy purposes. In this procedure, a 1 in 100 dilution of ammonium oxalate solution is made with the blood sample taken in ethylenediaminetetra acetic acid (EDTA) anticoagulant. This solution lyses the erythrocytes while preserving the platelets. Charge the counting chambers and wait for 15 minutes to the platelets to settle and count the platelets using 40× objective and count all the 25 small squares in the central of the chamber. Write down the results as platelets counted $\times 10^{3\mu l}$cells.

ERROS ASSOCIATED WITH MANUAL CELL COUNTS

They errors associated with manual cell counts are technical and inherent.

Technical errors can be minimised by avioding the following:

- Poor technique in obtaining the blood sample.
- Insufficient mixing of the blood sample
- Inaccurate pipetting and the use of badly calibrated pipettes or counting chambers.
- Inadequate mixing of the cell suspension
- Faulty filling of the counting chamber
- Careless counting of cells within the chamber

INHERENT ERRORS

This result from uneven distribution of cells in the counting chamber, and no amount of mixing will minimise this inherent variation in numbers between áreas. Inherent error can only be reduced by counting more cells in a preparation.

HOW TO PERFORM PLATELET COUNT ESTIMATION

The platelet estimate is performed under the 100× oil immersion objective lens. In an área of the blood film where the red blood cells barely touch, count the number of platelets and perform the average count of 10 fields.Multiply the average cells counted by 20,000, this approximates the platelet count. A rough guide states that when there are 7 to 25 platelets per oil immersion field, the platelet count is adequate provided there are approximately 200 red blood cells per oil immersion camp or field.In an anaemic condition, this does not hold true so a more involved formular may be used.

Platelet estimate:<u>Average number of platelet /field × Total Red cell count</u>

200 Red blood cells/Field

PERIPHERAL BLOOD MORPHOLOGY

Examination of the peripheral blood films are of utmost importance to the diagnosis of diseases. In addition to providing information about quantitative changes in blood cells, careful analysis of the quantitative changes may help in elucidating the underlying reasons for the clinical problems. These observations may identify the cause of anaemia or undiagnosed fever or the presence of a haemoglobinopathy. When glass slides are in short supply, laboratories sometimes find it necessary to wash and reuse slides.

MODIFIED (ONE-TUBE) OSMOTIC FRAGILITY TEST

This simple and inexpensive test for screening for β-Thalassaemia trait is useful when quantification of haemoglobinA$_2$ is not possible and standardised automated analysers are not available for accurate measurement of haematological índices (MCV, MCH and MCHC). A variety of concentrations of buffered saline have been used. A concentration of 0.36% in buffered saline is recommended to ensure a high sensitivity with an acceptable specificity. Because the false positive rate is around 10%, confirmation of a positive result requires referral of a sample to a laboratory able to quantitate haemoglobinA$_2$. The test can also be used to screen for α^0- Thalassaemia trait , with positive samples being referred to a reference centre for DNA molecular analysis. About 50% of samples containing haemoglobinE also give a positive result, this is an advantage because the detection of haemoglobinE is important in predicting the possibility of thalassaemia major or intermédia in compound heterozygotes with β –thalassaemia.

HAEMOGLOBIN E SCREENING TEST

Ideally, the diagnosis of haemoglobin E heterozygosity or homozygosity should be by haemoglobin electrophoresis at alkaline PH or High performance liquid chromatography(HPLC) with a second method being used to confirm the provisional identification. When these facilities are unavailable, a screening test using the blue dye, 2,6-Dichlorophenolindophenol (DCIP) can be used. Samples containing haemoglobin E become faintly turbid when incubated with DCIP.

Chapter-5

<u>LABORATORY SUPPORT FOR MANAGEMENT OF HIV/AIDS: CD4-POSITIVE T-CELL COUNTS</u>

Facilities for CD4- positive counts are essential in countries with a high incidence of HIV/AIDS, both for diagnosis and for identifying and monitoring patients who would benefit from antiretroviral therapy. A method using a simple low – cost single platform flow cytometer is now available and suitable for district hospital laboratories. However, it may still be too complex to maintain and too expensive for peripheral facilities in some economic distressed countries. A field friendly enzyme linked immunosorbent assay (ELISA) technique for quantifying CD4 – positive cells on dried blood spots has been described. However, it is not yet confirmed whether this method is effective for samples with low CD4+ counts. Other methods including dipstick systems are being developed and still require field trials.

LABORATORY MANAGEMENT

INTERLABORATORY COMMUNICATION

A well planned logistical service is necessary to facilitate flow of communication between remote clinics and central laboratories and clinical consultants. This enables reports on specimens received from the periphery and relevant advice on diagnosis and patient management to be sent without delay from the central laboratory to the periphery. The major delay in test turn around time is the result of slow delivery of reports after the test has been performed. Telefax and e-mail facilities have helped to eliminate this delay, but they are dependent on fixed line communications and electrical supplies, both of which are frequently absent at remote rural clinics.

A potential solution is the use of a digital wireless data communications system such as the global system of mobile (GSM) network for laboratory reporting. In some economically distressed countries,rural populations have Access to wireless comunications that are relatively well maintained. The data volume required for text based laboratory reports is extremely modest and their transmission is low cost. Result reporting can either be incorporated into the mainstream laboratory information system or by individual handsets for smaller independent laboratories.

SPECIMEN TRANSPORT

The special problem of transporting specimens from remote clinics to laboratories and reference centres requires further consideration. Relatively well equiped peripheral laboratories can assist in rural development initiatives by creating employment opportunities for bicycle riders, motorcyclists, táxi operators, formal and informal courier companies and even helicopter service providers.

STAFF TRAINING

In poorer countries, there is often no system for regular supervision of an individuals´performance in the laboratory and many staff do not receive continuing Professional development. Monitoring standards of practice should continue for the whole Professional life of the laboratory technologist to ensure high quality results. However, because anaemia is the most prevalent disorder worldwide and is often the first sign of underying disease, the importance of reliable Hb estimation cannot be over stressed. This continuing education should include the whole range of tests offered by the laboratory and not only tests that are used to support the diagnosis of specific diseases.

Individuals need to keep their own training records, perhaps in the form of a log book, and to have their training achievements and plans regularly reviewed by their line managers. Central records of all training should also be maintained for monitoring purposes and to ensure equitable and appropriate distribution of training between different levels of staff. Regular monitoring of the quality of results from individual laboratories will enable specific problems to be identified and issues such as equipment failures, discontinuity of supplies and communication breakdowns should be brought to the attention of regional management teams.

CLINICAL STAFF INTERACTION

Appropriate clinical use of the laboratory has a direct impact on the cost effectiveness of the service. Laboratory tests may be initiated by nurses, health field workers and public health officers as well as medical doctors. Many of these persons have little or no technical training in how to request appropriate tests, how to provide timely and suitable samples and how to use the results for maximal benefit to the patients. Training for laboratory users needs to be incorporated into laboratory training programmes and closely monitored. In poorer countries, there is often a dearth of clinicians with both clinical and laboratory experience who are qualified to provide such training. Under these circumstances, the relationship between the laboratory and clinical staff can be enhanced and use of the laboratory can be optimised by using a clinician / technologist team to provide joint training in both disciplines.

HEALTH MANAGEMENT TEAMS

Local health management teams are often responsible for ensuring that their laboratories are provided with the necessary tools to deliver high quality service. As a rule, these teams do not include members of the laboratory profession who are only represented by other allied professionals such as pharmacists. Staff in economically destressed laboratories, are therefore not always responsible for purchasing supplies and equipment for the laboratory and this results in wastage through the purchase of inappropriate or poor quality equipment and reagents. Inaddition to encouraging adequate representation of laboratory professionals at management level, it is important to ensure that non laboratory personnel responsible for making decisions about economic destressed laboratories are educated about the needs of their laboratory service.

HEALTH AND SAFETY

Awareness of health and safety should be constantly promoted within all laboratories and the working environment needs to be made as safe as possible. A code of safe laboratory practice should be prepared that is affordable and relevant to the local circumstances. It should include the following:

> - Risk assessment – identification of the potential workplace hazards and the risk they pose to individuals working or visiting the laboratory.
> - Education on safe working practices.
> - Monitoring of adherence to health and safety regulations.
> - Prompt reporting and investigation of laboratory accidents.

Disposable syringes are intended for single use only. They cannot withstand sterilisation and should never be reused. Similarly, disposable lancets for skin puncture must never be reused. The practice of using a single lancet on several patients consecutively and cleaning it with alcohol between use is totally unacceptable.

REFERENCES

1. Faiz MA, Yunus EB, Rahman MR et tal 2002: Failure of national guidelines to diagnose uncomplicated malária in Bangladesh. American journal of tropical medicine and hygiene 67:396-399.
2. Akpek G, Lee SM, Gagnon DR et tal 2001:Bone marrow aspiration, biospy and culture in evaluation of HIV- infected patients for invasive mycobacteria and histoplasma infections. American Journal of Haematology 67:100-106.
3. Sherman GG, Galpin JS, Patel JM et tal 1999: CD4+ T cell enumeration in HIV infection with limited materials. Journal of immunological methods 222:209-217.
4. Glencross DK, Mendelow BV, Stevens WS et tal 2003: Laboratory monitoring of HIV/AIDS in a resource poor setting. South African medical Journal 93:262-263.
5. World Health Organisation 1998: Laboratory services for primary health care: Requirements for essential clinical laboratory tests ,Documents:LAB/98.1., WHO Geneva.
6. Mundy CJF,Bates I et al 2003: The operation , quality and costs of a district hospital laboratory service in Malawi. Transactions of the royal society of tropical medicine and hygiene 97:403-408.
7. Lewis SM, Stott GJ, Wynn KJ et tal 1998: An inexpensive and reliable new Haemoglobin colour scale for assessing anaemia. Journal of clinical pathology 51:21-24.
8. Van Den Broek NR, Ntonya C, Mhanga E et tal 1999: Diagnosing anaemia in pregnancy in rural clinics:assessing the potential of the Haemoglobin colour scale. Bulletin of the World Health Organisation 77:15-21.
9. Monstresor A, Ramsan M, Khalfan N et tal 2003: Performance of the Haemoglobin colour scale in diagnosing severe and very severe anaemia. Tropical Medicine International Health 8:1-6.
10. World Health Organisation 2000: Recommended methods for the visual determination of white blood cell count and platelet count: Document WHO/DIL/00.3. WHO Geneva.
11. Kattamis C, Efremov G, Pootrakul S 1981: Effectiveness of one tube Osmotic fragility screening in detecting β- thalassaemia trait. Journal of medical Genetics 18:266-270.
12. Chapple L, Harris A, Phelan L et tal 2005: Reassessment of a simple chemical method using DCIP for screening Haemoglobin E. Journal of clinical pathology 59:74-76.
13. Mwaba P, Cassol S, Pilon R, et tal 2003: Use of dried whole blood spots to measure CD4+ Lymphocyte counts in HIV-1 infected patients. Lancet 362:1459-1460.